"There is no greater agony than bearing an untold story inside you."
— Maya Angelou

After the Injection

A Memoir of Survival and Resistance

By

Angeline Moyo

(née Ndebele)

After the Injection: A Memoir of Survival and Resistance

Published in the United States

Legal Disclaimer

This is a work of nonfiction based on the author's lived experience. All events are portrayed as truthfully and accurately as memory allows. However, in some instances, names, dates, locations, and identifying details have been changed or obscured to protect the privacy of individuals and comply with legal and ethical obligations. The views expressed in this memoir are those of the author alone and do not reflect the opinions of any medical, legal, or governmental institution. The content is not intended as medical advice and should not be relied upon as a substitute for professional care or clinical treatment. The author does not accept any liability for the use or misuse of the information contained in this memoir

General Disclaimer

This memoir is a personal account based on the lived experiences of the author, Angeline Moyo. It reflects her memories, interpretations, and emotions surrounding the events she endured as a nurse, psychiatric patient, and survivor of systemic injustice. In order to protect the privacy and confidentiality of individuals, all names of healthcare professionals and institutions have been changed or anonymised. While every effort has been made to present events truthfully, this book is not intended to serve as a clinical, legal, or diagnostic account. It is not a substitute for medical advice, nor does it claim to represent the experiences of all patients, nurses, or mental health professionals. Some scenes and conversations have been reconstructed from memory and may be approximated for narrative clarity. The author acknowledges that others involved may remember events differently.

Trigger Warning

This memoir contains detailed accounts of psychiatric hospitalization, forced medication, suicide attempts, racism, medical negligence, and institutional abuse. These themes may be distressing for some readers, particularly those with lived experience of trauma, mental illness, or systemic injustice. Please care for your well-being as you read. Take breaks as needed, and seek support if you find any part of this narrative overwhelming.

Author's Note on Purpose

After Injection: A Memoir of Survival and Resistance is a deeply personal account of my journey through mental illness, forced psychiatric treatment, racial injustice, and recovery. I write as a survivor, a nurse, a mother, and a Black African woman navigating a mental health system that often silences those it claims to help.

This memoir is not written to assign blame to individuals, but to challenge the structures and attitudes that perpetuate harm. It is a call for empathy, accountability, and transformation in how we understand and respond to mental distress—especially when experienced by people of colour, migrants, and professionals.

My intention is to honour truth, ignite conversation, and encourage others who have been silenced to find their voice. While this story reflects my unique experience, I know it echoes the lives of many who remain unheard. This book is for them.

Table of Contents

Introduction:

When the Healer Breaks

My name is Angeline. I was born and raised in Zimbabwe, in a rural village where life was simple but hard. We lived close to the land—planting, harvesting, fetching water, cooking over open fire. We didn't have much in terms of material things, but we had structure, faith, and family. My mother was a quiet, strong woman. My father was strict but dependable. There were many of us—siblings, cousins, aunties—all in the same space. Community raised us.

From a young age, I was drawn to caregiving. I helped nurse younger siblings through fevers, cleaned wounds with boiled water and herbs, and sat with elders when they were sick. I saw the strength of the women in my family—how they bore pain without complaint, how they held everything together even when they were falling apart. But I also saw something else. A shadow. A silence.

My maternal grandmother died by suicide before I was born. It was barely spoken of—just a whisper behind closed doors. Later on, my younger brother would take his life too, at the age of 24. I didn't know then how deeply this legacy of unspoken pain would shape me.

Education was the way out. I was determined to become a nurse—not just because I loved caring, but because it was one of the few professions where a Black African woman could gain respect, stability, and a measure of independence. I earned my diploma in nursing and worked in hospitals back home. But like many others, I dreamed of going abroad—of making more money, seeing more of the world, sending something back to my family.

In September 2001, I left Zimbabwe and came to the UK. It was both exciting and terrifying. I arrived with hope, a head full of knowledge, and a heart ready to serve. I believed that here, in this modern country, my skills would be valued. That if I worked hard, I would be respected.

I never imagined that I would one day find myself as a patient in a locked ward, fighting not just for my life—but for my right to be seen as human.

My journey through the NHS began in June 2002 at a rehabilitation hospital. I started as a junior nurse, determined to prove myself through hard work.

From early on, I noticed that not everyone was treated the same. I saw how white English nurses were favoured, how Black African nurses were often overlooked, spoken down to, or accused of being "too loud" or "too slow." At first, I told myself it didn't matter—I would prove myself. I would rise through hard work.

In 2005, eager to deepen my knowledge, I began a self-sponsored nursing degree, which I completed in 2008. That September, I stepped into a new role as a shift leader in an acute stroke unit—a job that should have marked a new beginning.

Instead, it marked the start of an invisible war.

Almost immediately, I encountered insubordination and hostility from some white English nurses on the unit. Their resistance wasn't about clinical disagreements or protocol—it was personal. Subtle undermining. Refusals to follow direction. Whispered comments that stung in their precision.

I did what I had been taught to do: I followed the correct reporting channels and raised the issue with the ward manager. But no action was taken. My concerns dissolved into silence.

In August 2009, I was abruptly moved from the acute unit to the stroke rehabilitation unit without consultation. It was a demotion masked as a transfer—one that stripped me of responsibility and erased my leadership role without explanation. The message was clear: *You do not belong.*

A month later, while covering a night shift as an agency nurse in a different unit, tragedy struck. A patient unexpectedly passed away at the very start of my shift. Grief came fast and loud—the parents erupted in anger and disbelief. I was blamed for failing to manage the situation, even though the death had preceded any medical input I could have offered. A white English male colleague made false allegations about my conduct that night. Once again, I found myself at the centre of suspicion, not support.

I was suspended for three months pending an investigation. The process was flawed from the start. The investigator was not impartial; his bias was visible in the way he conducted the inquiry. Key witnesses were not included. He dismissed my explanations and leaned into the false narrative constructed against me.

Through the Trust grievance procedure, I formally complained about the racism I had endured. To my surprise and disappointment, my voice was muted by bureaucracy. My complaints were neither acknowledged nor addressed.

Disciplinary actions followed relentlessly. The matron eventually moved me to a clinical area where I had no prior experience—another tactic to destabilize and demoralize me.

By 2011, I knew I had to leave bedside nursing for the sake of my own wellbeing. I enrolled in a Human Resource Management course at a university, self-funded. I thought education would take me in a new direction.

I reduced my hours to part-time, thinking I might find some reprieve. Instead, I was met with even more pressure. The workload was unbearable, the expectations punitive.

In January 2012, I could no longer take it. I resigned from the NHS—not because I was unfit or unwilling, but because the environment had become toxic. It was constructive dismissal, shaped by racism, undermining, and emotional exhaustion. I left with dignity, but also with deep wounds.

I initiated legal proceedings against my former employer. It was a bold move, driven by a deep need for justice and recognition. But just a week before my tribunal date, my solicitor withdrew from the case. I was left without legal representation and couldn't find another in time. The tribunal was cancelled. I felt abandoned—not just by the system, but by the very structures that were supposed to protect workers like me.

I joined a nursing agency part-time while continuing with my HR studies. But even in agency work, the pattern repeated. I was just another "Black nurse" on the rota—disposable and disrespected.

In 2015, I stopped working altogether. By 2016, I had completed my HR course, but I couldn't bring myself to apply for jobs. My confidence had been shattered. I felt like a failure.

Between 2016 and 2019, I stayed at home. I was deeply demotivated. I didn't know it at the time, but I was already slipping into the grip of depression. The years of fighting, enduring, and being silenced had all built up.

By the summer of 2019, I was exhausted—mentally, emotionally, and physically. After years of being overlooked, overworked, and mistreated, I had lost my motivation, my energy, and my sense of direction. I was deeply withdrawn, emotionally flat, and unable to see any light ahead. But I was not suicidal. I delayed looking for work in HR, paralyzed by doubt. *Was I good enough? Would I be accepted in a new field?* Each day that passed added to my sense of failure. I wasn't just unemployed—I felt invisible.

In August 2019, my husband, noticing my low mood and emotional decline, referred me to the local mental health crisis team. He told them I was unwell.

They didn't assess me. They didn't listen to me. They listened only to him. They arranged for me to be detained under Section 2 of the Mental Health Act—for up to 28 days—for "assessment and treatment."

It was the beginning of a journey I never imagined: from nurse to psychiatric patient.

At the hospital, my identity and experience as a healthcare professional seemed to vanish. I wasn't treated as someone with decades of knowledge and training—I was seen only as a Black, middle-aged woman with a "mental illness." I had never experienced hallucinations or delusions. My symptoms were consistent with depression, not psychosis. But my protests were dismissed.

I was admitted without an individual assessment. The admitting doctor never spoke with me directly. Instead, he took the crisis team's account at face value, filled in the paperwork from his office, and prescribed antipsychotic medication without any dialogue. That night, when the nurse came to give me the tablets, I refused. Something in me resisted the injustice, even in my broken state.

The next day, I was informed of my right to appeal the detention through a tribunal. I held onto that right like a lifeline and submitted the application the same day. The hearing was set for three weeks later.

In those weeks, I continued to refuse the tablets. But the system found another way to assert control. Without my consent, a depot injection of antipsychotic medication was prescribed. I was restrained and injected in an undignified and traumatic manner. A week later, it happened again—the same injection, the same violation of my body and autonomy.

When the tribunal finally convened, it ruled in my favour. But the system failed me again: I was sent home without a discharge care plan, without community support, and still under the heavy chemical influence of a drug I should never have received.

Two weeks after the injection, I began to deteriorate rapidly. My thinking slowed. My emotions dulled. My body felt foreign.

I felt the full weight of what had happened. I was physically and mentally unwell. I went to my GP, who diagnosed me with depression and prescribed antidepressants. I took them for a month with no improvement. Instead, I sank deeper. Suicidal thoughts became a constant companion.

I returned to the GP, who referred me to a community psychiatrist. The appointment was set for the 10th of February 2020—nearly three months away.

But I didn't make it to that appointment.

Chapter One:

Cracks in the Foundation

"Trauma is not what happens to us, but what we hold inside in the absence of an empathetic witness."
— PETER A. LEVINE

In 2012, something inside me began to shift—a quiet unravelling that no one, not even I, fully understood at the time. After years of dedication to my role as a general nurse and shift leader in a demanding hospital ward, I reached a breaking point. The pressure became unbearable. I felt unsupported, isolated, and overwhelmed. Eventually, I made the difficult decision to leave. Though it was framed as my resignation, in my heart I knew it was constructive dismissal. I felt forced out—pushed by a system that expected too much and gave too little in return.

Still determined to find a new path, I took on part-time agency nursing work after resigning from my NHS job and enrolled in a Human Resource Management course at university. I also initiated legal proceedings against my former employer. It was a bold move, driven by a deep need for justice and recognition. But just a week before my tribunal date, my solicitor withdrew from the case. I was left without legal representation and couldn't find another in time. The tribunal was cancelled. I felt abandoned—not just by the system, but by the very structures that were supposed to protect workers like me.

I pressed on with my studies, pouring my energy into education. In 2016, I completed the HR course. But instead of feeling accomplished, I felt lost. I stopped working in nursing altogether and allowed my professional registration to lapse. I stayed home, drifting in a fog of exhaustion and disillusionment. The transition from being a caregiver to someone without a clear role in the world was disorienting. My confidence crumbled. Family relationships began to suffer under the weight of my unspoken distress.

I delayed looking for work in HR, paralyzed by doubt. Was I good enough? Would I be accepted in a new field? Each day that passed added to my sense of failure. I wasn't just unemployed—I felt invisible.

By August 2019, my emotional state had deteriorated significantly. After suffering from a cold for a week, I developed ringing in my right ear. At the time, my husband and I were not speaking. Instead of trying to understand what was troubling me—or involving a family counsellor—my husband contacted the local mental health crisis team. Without assessing me directly, they relied solely on his account. I was taken from my home and admitted under Section 2 of the Mental Health Act—a legal power allowing for forced hospitalization. I had no say.

Being sectioned felt like a storm had swept me into an alien world, where my voice was silenced before I even had a chance to speak. I was no longer Angeline Moyo—a nurse, a mother, a human being. I was reduced to a set of risks and labels, defined not by careful clinical observation, but by hearsay and presumption. That erasure of identity cut deeper than any diagnosis ever could.

When I arrived at the hospital, I was composed and oriented. I still believed someone would assess me fairly. I expected a psychiatrist to sit with me, listen to my story, ask questions, and understand. Instead, the admitting doctor stayed in the ward office, writing notes based on second-hand information and prescribing antipsychotic medication I didn't need.

I refused the medication. It didn't make sense. No one had explained what was happening or why. When I learned that I could appeal to a tribunal, I applied immediately. But while I waited, I was placed under constant observation. I wasn't violent. I wasn't shouting. I wasn't a danger to anyone. I was just deeply unhappy—but I remained composed.

Within two days of my admission, I was summoned to meet with the psychologist. I remember walking into that small, windowless room with walls the colour of old porridge and a chair too straight for comfort. My palms were clammy. I was still adjusting to the new rhythm of the ward—timed meals, locked doors, and the quiet hum of unspoken grief floating through the corridors.

But this room felt different. The psychologist, a woman in her late thirties with a calm face and a notepad that never left her lap, invited me to sit. And for once, someone asked me—not just how I felt—but what had happened.

So I told her.

I spoke for what felt like hours. My voice trembled at first, but as the words poured out, they gathered strength. I told her how things had broken down between my husband and me—not suddenly, but in slow, painful fragments. Our marriage had once been built on youthful promises, but now it resembled a cold truce held together by obligation and silence. He didn't believe in my Human Resource Management studies, and I didn't believe in the funeral business he had started in Zimbabwe. Our dreams clashed, unacknowledged and unresolved.

Then I told her about the NHS. About the way I had been slowly suffocated by bullying—how my confidence was chipped away by colleagues who saw my strength as a threat. I had dedicated years to my nursing career, and yet I had been pushed out, dismissed without compassion. It wasn't just a job I lost—it was a part of my identity.

The psychologist sat quietly, listening. Encouraging. And so I kept going.

I told her about growing up in a family of nine children—six girls and three boys—in rural Zimbabwe. I was the fifth child, a girl among many, and the only one who dared to go beyond primary school. Education had been my rebellion. When Maqhekeni Secondary School opened in 1984, I became one of its first students. We were the pioneers—the dreamers in dusty shoes.

I had no desk, no textbooks of my own. But I had hunger—the kind that doesn't fade with food. Jane, my closest friend, and I were so determined that the headteacher invited us to live with him at the teacher's cottage to shorten our daily walk. It was a kindness I never forgot.

When Jane transferred to a better school, I followed her path, moving to Madlambudzi Secondary School. It was tougher there—bigger, more competitive. I lived with relatives who made it clear that school was not their priority. I was worked hard—scrubbing, cooking, fetching water—my books forgotten under piles of chores.

Afraid of failing, I asked the headteacher, Mr. Gowero, for help. He offered me a place in his cottage. There, I found refuge again—until one Friday evening, when the biology teacher asked me to carry books to his room. I had no reason to fear him. But once I entered the room, he followed me in and locked the door behind him. What happened next took my voice, my innocence, my sense of safety.

He raped me.

There was a police camp nearby, but I didn't report it. I didn't believe anyone would protect me. In Zimbabwe, I had heard too many stories of girls being blamed, laughed at, or interrogated until they wished they had stayed silent. I told no one. He continued to teach me biology as if nothing had happened. I buried it and carried on.

Somehow, I passed my final exams. No one from my old school did. I qualified for A-Levels, but my family couldn't afford them. So I took a temporary teaching job, became the breadwinner for my parents and younger siblings, and carried their futures on my back—though none followed the path I had carved.

Teaching brought me joy, but not stability. I tried to get into a teacher's training college, but tribalism and nepotism blocked my way. So I pivoted. I applied to train as a nurse at a Catholic mission school—Brunapeg. That's where my path took root again. I qualified as a State Certified Nurse and was posted to a rural clinic with no doctor, no electricity, and too many patients.

It was during this time that I had my son with my boyfriend—soon to become my husband. We married a year later and had our daughter four years after that. I later returned to complete further nurse training, this time leaving my children with their father at the military quarters. I had met him at Madlambudzi. He had joined the army after school. Ours was never a perfect love. We stayed together for the sake of appearances, for our children, for the story we once believed in.

Then I told her about Caesar.My brother. My beautiful, gentle Caesar.

He was only 24 when he came back from South Africa and hanged himself near our rural home. The memory still guts me. My husband had been the last person to see him alive and handled the funeral arrangements. I never got to ask the questions that haunted me. His death broke something in me I didn't know was still intact.

When I finished speaking, I felt both drained and strangely lighter. The psychologist nodded and said she would make a note of our conversation in my file.

I hadn't expected what followed.

My story—this tapestry of loss, resilience, silence, and survival—was reduced to clinical shorthand. The ringing in my right ear, a symptom of tinnitus I'd lived with for years, was interpreted as auditory hallucinations. The justified anger I had expressed toward my husband—a reflection of deep emotional pain—was recorded as paranoia. No nurse came to ask for clarification. No one returned to talk.

Instead, the whispers began.

"She was sacked from her job," they murmured. "She bought a coffin for herself."

It was as if my truth had been fed into a machine and spat back out as madness. I had entrusted the system with my pain, and it had twisted it into pathology.

They did not see me.

Not as a woman.
Not as a mother.
Not as a survivor.

They saw only a diagnosis.

And the label they gave me—psychosis, danger, non-compliant—allowed them to act with force.

I was forcibly injected with Clopixol, a powerful antipsychotic, while restrained in full view of other patients. No one warned me of side effects. No one treated me with dignity. The following week, the same thing happened—my body violated, my autonomy erased. The cumulative effect of those injections was devastating. My mind slowed. I felt a fog settle over me, thick and suffocating.

The tribunal was set for the 12th of September. The panel ruled in my favour. I was discharged without even a parting conversation with a doctor or nurse. I simply walked out the doors, more broken than when I had entered.

Two weeks later, I began to unravel. I was physically weak and mentally fractured. It felt like the right side of my brain had stopped working. I went to my GP, who diagnosed me with depression and prescribed Citalopram. But the medication made things worse. Suicidal thoughts crept in—slow and steady. I returned to the GP, who referred me to a psychiatrist. The appointment was scheduled for three months later.

Chapter Two:

Through the System

"The system isn't broken. It was built this way."
— MICHELLE ALEXANDER

On the morning of February 3rd, 2020, I awoke with the overwhelming feeling that the world no longer had space for me. I didn't want to exist. I didn't want to die violently. I just wanted to disappear. But instead, I shattered everything.

My husband had gone out to the garage to work on his car. When he returned, he lay down on the sofa and fell asleep. I looked at him and felt something inside me break. Quietly, I went to the kitchen and swallowed every antidepressant I had, along with a handful of paracetamol. But what followed wasn't just a suicide attempt.

I picked up a heavy kitchen mortar and struck my husband on the head.

I don't remember what I felt—only a terrifying numbness, as if I had stepped outside my own body.

My two adult children, who were upstairs, heard the noise. My daughter came down first and found her father unconscious. She called 999. Paramedics arrived quickly and rushed him to the hospital, working to revive him.

Meanwhile, I was handcuffed and taken to the police station, barely aware of my surroundings. The overdose had left me drowsy, unsteady, and confused. I struggled to answer questions. The officers noticed my condition, but no one seemed to ask whether I had tried to take my own life. Their focus was entirely on what I had done to someone else.

After the initial questioning, I was taken to a changing room. There, I was stripped of everything—my clothes, my dignity, and the last traces of my identity. I was handed a pair of prison-issue underpants and a thin t-shirt. I never saw my own clothes again. Then I was led into a cold, bare cell with nothing but a thin mattress and a single blanket.

The moment I lay down, I sank into a drug-induced sleep. Part of me hoped I would never wake up.

But I did.

Sometime in the night, I woke up disoriented. The grey walls around me felt like a nightmare, but the aching in my body reminded me it was all real. As the fog of medication lifted, so did the memory of what had happened. A sharp wave of anger and despair surged through me. Had my husband survived? I didn't know. There was no one to ask. I was alone—in every possible sense of the word.

I noticed a spare t-shirt in the cell and, in a moment of utter hopelessness, tore it apart. I wanted to strangle myself. I couldn't bear the shame or the thought that I might have killed someone I loved. A prison guard, hearing the tearing fabric, rushed over. He took the t-shirt away and threatened to strip me naked if I continued.

I was thirsty. My body, overwhelmed with toxins, felt heavy and sluggish. When I asked for water, it came in a tiny plastic cup. I didn't have the energy to ask for more.

After two days in police custody, I was taken to court—still handcuffed, still in prisoner's clothes. I was freezing. Standing before the judge, I heard the words *attempted murder* for the first time. It was surreal, like listening to someone else's story. I hadn't told anyone that I had tried to take my own life too. No one knew this was supposed to be my end as well.

I was remanded into custody and transferred to Foston Hall Prison in Derby—a place I had never even heard of. The journey there was silent. I shared the prison van with other women, but no one spoke. Each of us was locked inside our own shame and fear.

At the prison, we were processed. Health checks. Standard questions. Issued uniforms. By chance, I was given a single cell—most others had to share. I barely ate. I had no appetite and no desire to survive. Some officers noticed and brought food to my cell, but I often threw it away. I was trying to disappear.

I tore more t-shirts. I made more attempts to end my life. Still, no one asked why. It was only my refusal to eat that eventually drew concern. A prison nurse referred me to the mental health team. I didn't tell them I was suicidal. Instead, I said something felt wrong with the right side of my brain. I also mentioned the ringing in my right ear—something my GP had been investigating before everything happened. I'd already been diagnosed with partial hearing loss in that ear. The symptoms made me feel like I was unraveling from the inside out.

Eventually, I was referred to a visiting psychiatrist, Dr. Campbell. During our first meeting, I told him I believed the Clopixol injection had damaged my brain. He listened. He didn't dismiss me. He diagnosed me with severe depression and said I should be in a hospital, not a prison.

But I refused the transfer. I wanted to stay. I still hoped to starve myself to death.

Dr. Campbell prescribed antidepressants. I started taking them, not because I wanted to get better, but because I had no fight left in me. Six weeks later, despite my earlier refusal, I was transferred to a secure mental health hospital.

Once again, I was handcuffed and delivered to a locked facility. At reception, every item of clothing and every possession was inspected and logged. The staff were cold and indifferent. The nurse who searched me turned out to be the same one assigned to my ward. She gave me a tour and showed me to my room—another single cell.

It was lunchtime. I was led to the dining room, where other patients sat—some shouting, some silent, most somewhere in between. The atmosphere was tense, chaotic. The cutlery was plastic, the food served on small trays. I was handed a sandwich and ate without appetite.

The ward felt no different from prison—the same coldness, the same surveillance, the same sense of being judged. I sat alone in my room afterward, staring at the walls. My identity as a nurse had vanished. I wasn't a caregiver anymore. I was "a patient." A risk. A statistic.

While I was in prison, my son and daughter had kept in touch by phone. They even visited. They told me that on the day of the incident, they were removed from our home and placed in a hostel. The police had sealed off the house for a week, searching for evidence. They took the kitchen mortar, my laptop, and my phone. They said the items would be returned once the case was over. But they never were.

My children also told me their father was recovering in hospital. Knowing he had survived brought a strange mix of relief and guilt. I had hurt him. I had hurt them. My youngest daughter was away at university. I could only imagine how the news had shattered her world.

Now I was in a hospital—but not as a professional. Not as a healer. I was no longer the one offering comfort. I was the one in need. The shame was unbearable. The stigma, suffocating. My life, once ruled by shift patterns and patient charts, had spiraled into something unrecognizable.

And I had no control.
No voice.
Just time behind locked doors.

Chapter Three:

Life Behind the Locked Ward

"There is no greater sorrow than
to recall a time of joy in misery."
— DANTE ALIGHIERI

I was no longer a nurse. No longer a mother in her own home. No longer even a prisoner awaiting trial. I had entered a new category: mental health patient in a secure hospital. And though I already knew pain, humiliation, and loss, life behind the locked ward introduced a different kind of suffering—quiet, systematic, and soul-eroding.

The first few days passed in a blur. I attempted to take my own life several times, but each attempt was unsuccessful. Despite this, I was not placed on suicide watch. It was only one evening that a nurse, during routine checks, discovered a ligature made from a torn T-shirt around my neck. She escalated the incident immediately. From that night onward, I was placed on one-to-one suicide watch.

In that moment, my privacy and dignity were stripped away. With staff constantly stationed at my open door, I could barely sleep. I would lie in bed, staring at the staff as they sat nearby—some of them even dozing off during the night. I remained on suicide watch until my condition showed signs of improvement.

To my surprise, no one ever asked me why I was suicidal—not even the psychologist. I had several psychotherapy sessions, but none of them addressed the core of my distress. During one-to-one supervision, I tried to open up to the staff, hoping someone would listen to the truth. But no one seemed to want to hear it. Some dismissed my words as hallucinations. Others labelled me paranoid. A few even twisted and fabricated what I had shared.

The ward ran on a mechanical rhythm. Mornings began early with breakfast and medication rounds, followed by the daily ward meeting. But not everyone attended. In the acute ward, some patients were too unwell to participate, their silence speaking volumes.

Everything was controlled—when we ate, where we went, how long we could speak to family. Even the number of clothes we could receive and keep was counted. Every fragment of independence had to be negotiated or surrendered.

Each nurse wore a lanyard with keys that clinked like a constant reminder: freedom was out of reach.

The medication I had started in prison continued. I took the tablets, but they didn't seem to lift the fog. Instead, I felt more detached, more numb. I slept too long. My thoughts were slow and heavy. Sometimes I couldn't tell if it was the depression or the drugs causing the weight in my head. No one explained what the medications were really meant to do—just that I needed them. Just that I was "unwell."

I watched the other women. Some were loud and erratic. Others silent and broken. Many of us carried traumas like invisible luggage—abuse, abandonment, criminalisation. You could see it in our eyes. We were all here, but most of us didn't know how to begin healing.

Some staff tried to be kind, but kindness here was guarded, fleeting. Others treated us as cases to be managed, not people to be understood. I saw the strain—the shift patterns, the burnout. Some couldn't meet your gaze. Some spoke at you, not with you. It was a strange reversal: I had once worn the uniform. I had once stood on the other side. Now I was on the receiving end of silence, control, and institutional indifference.

Therapy was introduced slowly, and only when I was deemed "stable." But the sessions felt shallow. Sometimes I sat across from professionals and felt like a specimen. I tried to speak, but the words didn't always come. And when they did, I felt analysed for risk, not truly heard. They wanted to manage me, stabilise me—not see me.

During our first meeting, Dr. Campbell looked at me earnestly and said, "Angeline, you've spent years caring for others as a nurse. Now it's time to let someone care for you." His words sounded compassionate, but I was wary. I had already learned that kindness in these settings often came with conditions.

The antidepressants didn't help. My mood remained low, my mind fogged, my body foreign. The consultant tried different types, adjusted dosages, changed schedules. When nothing worked, he added an antipsychotic, explaining that NICE guidelines recommended this combination for treatment-resistant depression.

To my surprise, no one wanted to talk about the hospital that had forcibly injected me. No one acknowledged the system's role in my collapse. It was as if my trauma began and ended with that one violent act—ignoring the years of neglect and institutional injustice that led to it.

But slowly, something inside me began to stir. I found fragments of myself in writing. I kept a journal, scribbling thoughts, feelings, memories. I wrote because I needed to hear my own voice, even if no one else was listening. Writing became a lifeline—a place where I could exist without judgement.

It was in those pages that I began to process not only what had happened to me, but what had been done to me. I started to recognise the patterns—of racism, of misogyny, of psychiatric paternalism. I was not merely "ill." I had been wounded. And those wounds had been left to fester in silence.

Contact with my children was the only light. My son and daughter called and visited when they could. I could hear the worry in their voices, the heartbreak they tried to hide. They told me their father had survived and was recovering at home. That news brought relief, but also a deeper sorrow. I had hurt him. I had hurt them.

I often wondered how my youngest daughter—away at university—was coping. I hadn't spoken to her yet. The shame made it hard to imagine what she must have thought or felt. I had been her role model. Now I was behind locked doors, reduced to a shadow of the woman she knew.

Days passed slowly. I stared at the ceiling for hours, unable to sleep or think. I counted the steps from my bed to the door. I avoided conversation. Trust was hard to build in a place where everyone was trying to survive in their own way.

And yet, something shifted.

One night, I heard another patient crying softly. I didn't know her name, but I knew her pain. I wanted to tell her she wasn't alone.

And in that moment, I remembered who I was.

I remembered the nurse, the mother, the woman who had once been strong. That part of me wasn't gone. She was buried under grief, guilt, and exhaustion—but still alive. For the first time in a long time, I felt the faintest desire to fight for her again.

It wasn't hope—not yet. But it was the beginning of something.

Chapter Four:

Recovery and Resistance Behind Locked Doors

"When you can't change the system, refuse to let it change you."

After six months in the acute ward, I requested a transfer to a rehabilitation unit. I was relieved when my request was granted. Following an assessment, I was accepted. I knew the rehab ward would be quieter and more stable than the acute ward, and I needed that stillness. Around the same time, Dr. Campbell wrote to the court declaring that I was not fit to stand trial. My case was postponed.

The rehabilitation ward was nothing like the acute unit. There were no alarms ringing, no patients screaming through the night, no constant sense of crisis. It was calmer—still institutional, but with a trace of peace. Each patient had their own room, just like before, but now with a television. That small connection to the outside world felt grounding, even comforting.

There was a small kitchen for patients, and we could make tea whenever we wanted. It was a minor freedom, but after months of hot drinks being handed to us like medication, it felt like a meaningful act of autonomy. I continued with therapy, still carrying the weight of what had brought me here—but now with the mental space to begin reflecting.

At one point, we were allowed mobile phones and laptops. These became my lifeline. I started researching everything—especially the long-acting antipsychotic injection I had been given in 2019. I read medical journals, scanned patient forums, and studied NICE guidelines. I wanted to understand what had been done to my body and my mind. The side effects, the risks, my rights as a patient—it all mattered now in a way it hadn't before.

A few months into my time in rehab, Dr. Campbell resigned. Before leaving, he sent a letter to the Ministry of Justice declaring me fit to stand trial. That single letter would reshape the course of my stay.

He was replaced by Dr. Chapman, a temporary consultant on a three-month contract.

Despite everything, my children continued to visit. Their presence brought warmth and life back into a world that had grown sterile and cold. We were allowed one-hour visits that passed far too quickly. On one occasion, my husband came. Seeing him in person—seeing the scars on his head—was unbearable. The pain surged back through me like a flood. I was crushed under guilt and grief, and yet somehow still numb. I couldn't meet his eyes.

Each day on the rehab ward began at 8:00 a.m. with morning medication, followed by a daily ward meeting to discuss the structure of the day. Some patients had community leave, approved by the Ministry of Justice under Hospital Orders. I wasn't one of them. I was still considered high-risk. Until my trial was over, I wasn't allowed to step beyond the hospital walls.

In September 2020, I was finally given a court date.

That morning, I was handcuffed once again and transported in a hospital van. When I arrived, the sight of the courtroom—the jury, the judge, the legal staff—was overwhelming. I stood only to confirm my name, then sat and listened.

The prosecution played the video footage from the crime scene. I had never seen it before. I watched in disbelief, breath caught in my chest. They presented the case as attempted murder. There was no mention of my intent to take my own life. No real consideration of the mental health crisis that had spiralled out of control. No context. Just violence, stripped of meaning.

For reasons never fully explained, the judgment was delayed. Some hearings happened without me. I felt invisible. Powerless. When the judgment finally came, I was once again handcuffed, once again driven to court.

Dr. Chapman attended as the responsible clinician. My husband and two of my children were there. My daughter, who had been home during the incident, was called to give evidence. It must have been an impossible experience for her.

In the end, the court acknowledged my mental illness. The charge was amended—from attempted murder to "wounding." I was placed under a Hospital Order, meaning I would remain in secure care until I was deemed safe for release.

No prison sentence. But no freedom either.

The ruling came with legal restrictions on my movements. That judgment plunged me into a deep low. A sentence without a time limit feels like your life has been paused indefinitely. You can't breathe properly under the weight of it.

Around that time, a new consultant, Dr. Collins, was appointed on a permanent basis. He applied to the Ministry of Justice for me to be granted escorted leave outside the hospital. It was a slow and bureaucratic process—standard requests could take six weeks or more to receive a response. As with most new consultants, he also began reviewing my medications. At the time, I was on antidepressants and a low dose of an antipsychotic.

When I received that first permission to leave the hospital grounds, it felt like a small flame of hope had been lit. For the first time in years, I dared to believe that life outside those locked doors might still be possible.

My first walk was brief—just around the hospital grounds, escorted by two members of staff. It was such a simple thing, walking, yet it felt new and strangely awkward. My muscles had stiffened from months of confinement, and I tired quickly. Afterward, I would return to my room and lie down, rarely joining the others in the day area. I was still mentally recovering and trying to make peace with the reality of an indefinite Hospital Order. Staff interpreted my withdrawal as a sign of worsening depression and reported it to the consultant.

Dr. Collins told me she planned to increase both my antidepressants and antipsychotic medication. I tried to resist. I told her I wasn't depressed—I just needed time and space. But she insisted, citing NICE guidelines for treatment-resistant depression.

That decision changed my body—and my life.

Within weeks of starting the combined therapy, my appetite returned with force. I began eating well again, and soon the weight piled on. I went from 12 stone to 15 stone. But the weight gain came with other problems: I experienced shortness of breath with even minimal exertion, persistent back pain, and increased stiffness. A routine blood test revealed high blood sugar. I was diagnosed with Type 2 diabetes.

I tried to manage it through diet and exercise, even joined a local gym—but the weight kept climbing. I began to suspect that my medication was contributing to the problem. I challenged Dr. Collins about it. I told her the medication was doing more harm than good.

She believed in her diagnosis. I believed in my experience.

They treated the symptoms, but never the cause.

Then came the hearing loss in my right ear. A brain scan was ordered—it showed no significant changes. Still, my body was changing in ways that were alarming. But I kept going. I was no longer suicidal. I was determined to live, even in a body that no longer felt like mine.

Each year, I learned, the consultant submitted a report to the Ministry of Justice detailing my "attitude" toward medication. Those reports shaped my access to freedom. They had more power than the doctors ever admitted.

One day, I reached my limit.

I stopped swallowing the antipsychotic tablet. At the medication hatch, I'd pretend to take it, then return to my room and spit it into the sink. For a while, I got away with it. Until the day I forgot to flush. A cleaner found the tablet and reported it. The nurses identified it as mine and informed Dr. Collins.

She confronted me. I neither confirmed nor denied it. From then on, nurses were instructed to observe me for thirty minutes after each dose.

Still, I walked. Slowly, my strength returned.

I was allowed to go further—first to the local park with staff, then to nearby shops. Being in public again was intimidating. I felt exposed, as though people could see the invisible label stamped on me: "mentally ill," "criminal." But I walked anyway. I rested when needed. Then walked some more.

Eventually, I was trusted to leave the ward alone. I'll never forget that first solo outing. The wind touched my skin differently. I was free, if only for an hour. It was a precious step forward.

Back on the ward, routines ruled our lives. Morning meetings were mandatory. Missing one could cost you your leave for the day. But beyond the rituals, I began forming quiet friendships. Some patients had been there for years. We played Scrabble together. We shared laughter. We became real to each other, beyond diagnoses.

My children continued to visit regularly. Their visits were still supervised, still only an hour—but they were my light. Then came the day my husband visited.

Seeing him for the first time since the incident was heart-wrenching. The scars on his head were a stark, physical reminder of what had happened. I held myself together, but inside, I shattered all over again. By God's grace, he had recovered physically. But we both carried wounds deeper than skin.

Eventually, I was allowed to go out with my family to a restaurant—always with an escort present. But returning to our home remained forbidden. Even our conversations were monitored, often misunderstood by staff. I was no longer a wife, a mother, or a nurse. I was a risk to be managed.

Being reduced from a nurse to a psychiatric patient felt like being erased.

I remember when I first told Dr. Campbell that I wanted to request my old medical records from Hallam Street Hospital—the place where I had been given the Clopixol injection that changed everything. He looked at me and asked, "What are you going to do with that information?" He didn't expect me to act.

But under the Data Protection Act, I got those records.

What I found confirmed my worst fears: misinformation, fabricated assessments, and a lack of proper evaluation. The notes were a constructed narrative. The admitting doctor had copied information from the crisis team. The Black nurse who gave me the first injection claimed I gave consent. The white nurse who administered the second dose omitted the fact that I had been physically restrained.

The paperwork was neat. The boxes were ticked. The truth was buried. I filed a formal complaint with the NHS Trust three years later. The Chief Executive wrote back, saying an "independent" investigator had reviewed my case and found no wrongdoing. That investigator had never even spoken to me—she simply read the same biased paperwork and rubber-stamped the injustice.

When I pushed further, I was told to take my complaint to the Parliamentary and Health Service Ombudsman. I did. But they rejected it, saying I was out of time. I explained I had been mentally unfit during the one-year complaint window. They refused to make an exception.

Instead, they suggested a judicial review.

I contacted lawyers. Most of them dismissed my case. *"Psychological harm is not enough,"* they said. Others lost interest after seeing my bank statements. Judicial review, they reminded me, was expensive.

And so, the NHS Trust walked away unscathed.

I was left to carry the moral and psychological scars.

The one tool I had left was my mind—and my words. With access to a laptop and phone, I began researching. Connecting. Writing. That was when the seed for my first book was planted. I didn't want to tell my story as a victim. I wanted to bear witness.

A Black African nurse, punished for speaking up. Silenced by a system built to protect itself, not its patients.

I decided to name my book *White English Nurses Eat Black African Nurses*. The title came from a phrase I'd once heard from Judith Meissner, an American nursing professor: "*Nurses eat their young.*" I understood what she meant. But in my world, it wasn't just age or inexperience. It was race. Power. Institutional prejudice.

Through writing, I began to reclaim my strength. I realised that recovery wasn't just about pills and therapy sessions. It was about reclaiming my story. My truth. My voice.

It was about standing up, again and again, even when the system tried to keep me down.

Chapter Five:

A Silent Crisis

There is no greater sorrow than to recall happiness in times of misery — and to suffer in silence, unseen."
— DANTE ALIGHIERI

I can never forget that morning in April 2022. During our usual morning meeting, we received devastating news: one of the service users had taken her own life. She was only 23 years old.

While I was still in the acute ward, we had spent time together doing word searches. She had been studying for her A-levels and once told me she wanted to become a neurologist. She was incredibly bright, full of ambition and potential.

Her untimely death was a painful echo of my own past struggles. Like me, her suicide risk had been undocumented—she was not on suicide watch, only subject to routine checks. At one point, she had been preparing for discharge in the rehabilitation ward.

After an altercation with a staff member, she was moved back to the acute ward, though she still had permission for community leave to visit her parents.

I searched online for more information. According to her post-mortem report, she had been in hospital since 2017, and her mental health challenges had begun at the age of eleven.

For safety and privacy reasons, we were not told how she died. Staff only said she was found unresponsive during a routine check.

Her death stirred memories long buried within me—especially of my younger brother, who died by suicide at the age of 24. After his death, I never imagined I would one day also reach that dark edge, wanting to end my own life. Her passing reopened those wounds but also reignited my determination to understand the silent crisis that is suicide.

I began researching. I discovered that suicide can have a genetic component. In my own family, my maternal grandmother had taken her life before I was born, and a number of my cousins had also died by suicide.

My curiosity led me to the International Association for Suicide Prevention (IASP). I emailed them and requested more information. That's when I learned about World Suicide Prevention Day, observed every year on the 10th of September since 2003.

To my surprise, despite its global recognition, not many people—especially within the mental health services I'd encountered—seemed aware of this day. And yet, globally, suicide remains one of the leading causes of death.

Reflecting on my profession as both a nurse and a patient, I've seen how our healthcare system treats physical wounds with urgency, but emotional wounds are often met with discomfort, avoidance, or silence. Nowhere is that silence louder than around the topic of suicide.

I realized how little awareness, training, and open conversation there was around suicide prevention. It is often brushed aside in our practice, even though many patients are quietly suffering. This lack of recognition deepened my resolve to transform my pain into purpose.

I speak as someone who has stood at the edge of despair, when it felt like there was no one to turn to. From my lived experience, I now believe this truth: silence can kill—but speaking can heal.

People openly talk about heart disease, cancer, and diabetes without shame. So why is suicide different? Why is mental pain something we hide? Why do we only whisper about it after someone is gone?

Chapter Six:

Silent Struggles in the Caring Profession

"What hurts the victim most is not the cruelty of the oppressor but the silence of the bystander."
— ELIE WIESEL

The suicide of the young service user unsettled me deeply. Her death was not only a personal loss—it cracked open a door to deeper reflection on the broader issue of suicide, especially within the nursing profession. I began to ask myself serious questions: Why do so many nurses, trained to care for others, suffer in silence? Why is mental health still so overlooked in a profession built on compassion?

I started researching suicide among healthcare professionals and was disturbed by what I found. Nurses are disproportionately affected by suicide compared to many other professions. One study revealed that female nurses, in particular, are at significantly higher risk. I couldn't help but wonder how many of them, like me, had suffered quietly—battling unprocessed trauma, workplace bullying, institutional racism, and emotional burnout.

In my own journey, I had faced all of these. The emotional weight of feeling undervalued, dismissed, and discriminated against had slowly eroded my sense of self-worth. Even after the attempted murder-suicide and my long road through psychiatric treatment, it remained clear: the system often fails to recognize psychological pain until it is too late.

I began to feel a responsibility—not just to tell my story, but to shed light on this unspoken epidemic in nursing. As I dug deeper, I discovered advocacy organizations and professional bodies beginning to acknowledge the issue. Some hospitals were rolling out staff wellbeing programs. But many of these initiatives felt tokenistic—focused more on appearance than genuine change.

I read stories of nurses who, like me, had reached the edge. Some found their way back. Others didn't. One story stayed with me: a nurse in her forties who died by suicide after her formal complaint about bullying was ignored. She had been described as dedicated, compassionate, and deeply committed to her work. Her family and friends were shocked—but I wasn't. I understood the despair that could drive someone to that point.

It became painfully clear that part of the problem lies in the culture of healthcare itself. Nurses are expected to be resilient, selfless, endlessly giving. There is little space for vulnerability. Speaking up is often seen as weakness—or worse, insubordination. Those who raise concerns risk being labelled troublemakers, or even mentally unstable.

As a Black woman, the dynamics were even more complex. My attempts to speak out had been met with silence or punishment. My emotional distress was dismissed, my competence questioned, my survival reframed as aggression. The system had no language for my pain—no tools to understand or address the realities of my experience.

But I was no longer willing to be silenced.

I wanted to share my story, not as a tale of defeat, but as a call to action. I wanted other nurses to know: it's okay not to be okay. More importantly, we deserve to be heard, helped, and protected.

World Suicide Prevention Day—10th of September—must be recognized and honoured. From now on, I will mark it by writing a short blog post and sharing it on a mental health forum. That small act gives me hope. Perhaps change won't come overnight, but by breaking the silence, I'll be taking the first step.

I am reclaiming not just my voice, but my profession, my identity, and my power.

In the quiet of the rehabilitation ward, between therapy sessions and morning meetings, I began outlining this memoir. It was no longer just about survival—it was about transformation. And in the act of writing, I found a new purpose: to speak the truth others are afraid to say, and to honour those who never had the chance to speak at all.

Chapter Seven:

The Unseen Wound

"Just because no one else can heal or do your inner work for you doesn't mean you can, should, or need to do it alone."

— LISA OLIVERA

Looking back, I am certain of one thing: I was not suicidal before the forced Clopixol injection. What I was experiencing may be more accurately described as **Post-Traumatic Embitterment Disorder (PTED)**—a condition I later learned about through Christine Pratt's book *Silent Epidemic*. PTED affects individuals who have functioned well until they experience a profound injustice or trauma that shakes their psychological foundations. In my case, that trigger was not a single event but a series of violations: the inappropriate sectioning, the indifference of the system, and the forced administration of a powerful antipsychotic against my will.

Clopixol is a long-acting antipsychotic that binds strongly to dopamine D1 and D2 receptors. Dopamine plays a vital role in regulating motivation, emotion, and behaviour. Blocking it—especially in someone who is not psychotic—can result in anhedonia, emotional numbness, depression, and even suicidality. The injection didn't just sedate me. It silenced me. It dulled my mind, stiffened my body, and began to blur the edges of who I was. I remember trying to explain to the consultant that something was terribly wrong—that I felt as if my brain had been damaged. His response wasn't just dismissive. It was paternalistic, even mocking. When I requested access to my medical records, he asked, "What are you going to do with them?"

That moment changed everything. I realised this wasn't just a medical misjudgement—it was a systemic betrayal. My decline after the injection wasn't incidental. It was the direct consequence of a coercive medical act that ignored my history, my diagnosis, and most importantly, my voice.

The consequences weren't just psychological. I now live with hearing loss in my right ear—an unexplained side effect that emerged shortly after the injection. Though it's difficult to prove a direct connection, the timing is impossible to ignore. No other medical explanation has ever been offered.

What made the ordeal even more unbearable was the wall of institutional silence. I went through every official route available—the NHS Trust, the Care Quality Commission, the Parliamentary and Health Service Ombudsman—only to be met with bureaucracy, technicalities, and dismissal. My complaint was ruled "out of time." My injury was classified as "psychological," and thus not considered grounds for legal redress.

And yet I ask: what if the damage is neurological? What if trauma leaves marks that no MRI can detect, but which nevertheless shatter a person's sense of self?

Our system still clings to an outdated dichotomy—physical injuries matter, psychological ones don't. But psychological injuries can be just as devastating. They can steal your memory, your personality, your will to live. And when they are caused by the very system that claims to care, the harm is compounded.

We need to challenge how antipsychotic medications are used—especially when administered by force, and especially when the patient is not psychotic. We need to broaden our understanding of harm and stop ignoring invisible wounds simply because they don't show up on a scan.

As a nurse, I was trained to value patient-centred care. But this experience taught me that the system doesn't always honour that principle—especially when it views the patient as a problem to be controlled rather than a person to be heard.

Reflection

Being forcibly medicated with Clopixol changed me. Not just physically, but spiritually and emotionally. It taught me how fragile autonomy is when confronted with institutional power. It revealed how the line between care and harm can become dangerously blurred. What is called treatment can sometimes become a form of trauma.

And yet, it also revealed something else: resilience.

In speaking out, in writing this chapter, I begin the slow, painful, but necessary work of reclaiming my voice and asserting my truth. I may never receive justice for what happened, but I can insist that it be known. That it be named.

And perhaps—just perhaps—by telling my story, I will help to shift the system that so easily dismissed me.

Chapter Eight:

Overdue for Freedom

"Freedom is never voluntarily given by the oppressor; it must be demanded by the oppressed."
— MARTIN LUTHER KING JR.

By this stage of my journey, I had completed all the rehabilitative and educational programs required under my hospital order. I was stronger—physically, mentally, emotionally. I could walk to the farther shops alone, handle my own errands, and return without incident. I was no longer the fragile woman who once needed two escorts just to step beyond the hospital grounds.

And yet, despite my progress, one painful truth lingered: I was overdue for discharge.

A few months earlier, my consultant, Dr. Shay-Anne Pantall, had resigned. Before leaving, she assured me she would apply to the Ministry of Justice for permission to begin escorted visits home—a milestone for someone under a restricted hospital order. But for reasons never explained, the application was never submitted. Her departure left me in limbo.

A temporary female consultant was appointed for three months. She promised to pick up where Dr. Collins had left off. I allowed myself a flicker of hope. But once again, nothing moved forward. Her contract ended, and I was no closer to home.

Then came a new permanent consultant: Dr. Dickson. I had hoped that with some continuity, my situation might finally progress. But instead, the struggle simply changed shape. Having read the handover notes branding me "non-compliant" with medication, Dr. Dickson approached me with caution. He was hesitant to support my long-standing request to taper off the antipsychotic I had always maintained was unnecessary.

I pleaded with him. I asked not to be judged by old reports but to be seen for who I had become. I asked him to listen—not just to my case file, but to me. After several long and honest conversations, he agreed to a slow reduction of the medication, with the goal of discontinuation. It felt like a small victory. But it came at a cost: another bureaucratic wall.

Because I was under a restricted section, any changes to my medication plan, and any requests for unescorted leave, had to be approved by the Ministry of Justice. By then, I had been allowed to visit home for brief three-hour periods, but only under escort. I wanted the chance to prove that I could manage on my own.

Meanwhile, my mental health solicitor had submitted an application to the Ministry for my discharge through the Mental Health Tribunal. A date was set. For the first time in a long while, I had a glimmer of hope. Freedom felt within reach.

Then came the blow.

The Ministry of Justice rejected the application for unescorted leave. Without that crucial step, the Tribunal would likely find it too risky to discharge me directly into the community. The Ministry insisted I go to a monitored step-down placement, where my medication could continue to be supervised. I felt shackled all over again—not by my mental health, but by decisions made by officials who had never met me, who knew nothing of my progress.

Dr. Dickson told me candidly that, given the Ministry's rejection, he could not support a discharge home. A family meeting was arranged. My husband and children expressed their hope and readiness to have me back. But Dr. Dickson remained firm. Without the Ministry's endorsement, he could not endorse my release.

I had not posed a risk. I had shown no concerning behaviour since my admission. Yet none of it mattered.

On the morning of my Tribunal, Dr. Dickson met with my solicitor. His refusal to support my discharge left my legal team with no viable strategy. The hearing was cancelled. I was devastated—not only by the cancellation, but by the realization that the very consultant meant to advocate for my care had been rendered powerless. His authority was more symbolic than real. The Ministry of Justice held the reins.

In that moment, the illusion of patient-centred care collapsed. No matter how much insight I gained, how much progress I made, or how strong my support network was, the system would not release its grip.

Still, I held onto my resolve.

I had a life waiting for me—a home, a family, and an identity that stretched far beyond hospital walls. I had learned to live with my mental health history without shame. I knew now that being labelled with mental illness did not define me, just as it doesn't define the countless others who live in silence, without diagnosis or detention.

There are no blood tests or brain scans that can definitively measure a person's mental state. Psychiatry is not a hard science. And yet the system treats its diagnoses as if they are immutable truths.

Recovery, for me, is no longer about checking boxes set by bureaucrats. Recovery is about reclaiming my own narrative. It's about learning to live with dignity after being marked by stigma. It's about saying: *I am more than what was done to me.*

And no tribunal, no consultant, no ministry can take that away.

Chapter Nine:

Reclaiming My Voice

"I am no longer accepting the things I cannot change. I am changing the things I cannot accept."
— ANGELA DAVIS

The cancellation of my tribunal at the eleventh hour left me gutted—silenced yet again by a system that seemed engineered to suppress. That morning, I woke early, buoyed by hope. I took my time getting ready, carefully grooming myself not just for the day, but possibly for a new beginning. I told my peers I was going to my tribunal and might be discharged. They wished me luck. I felt a lightness I hadn't known in years.

My family arrived early to meet with the solicitor. My husband was prepared to give evidence, and my children were ready to speak—each of them hoping that this would finally be the moment we could live under one roof again. We believed this day would mark the end of our long separation.

But that fragile hope crumbled when the solicitor quietly pulled us aside. The tribunal would not go ahead. Dr. Dickson had refused to support my discharge, and without a consultant's backing, we stood no chance. The hearing was cancelled.

We sat together in the waiting room, stunned and silent. For nearly an hour, we tried to absorb the blow. The pain wasn't just mine—it radiated through my family. They had stood by me for five long years, clinging to hope. Now we faced a longer, more uncertain road.

Dr. Dickson proposed the "step-down" route—discharge into supported accommodation, where I would be monitored before being allowed home. To me, it felt like yet another rejection. Another barrier. Another institution between me and freedom.

Back on the ward, my peers gathered to hear how the tribunal had gone. I told them the truth: it never happened. They expressed sympathy, but soon our conversation shifted. Each of us was battling the same invisible machinery. In that moment, our shared frustrations forged a quiet, collective solidarity.

The Ministry of Injustice

Through this experience, I came to see the Ministry of Justice not as a guardian of fairness, but as an instrument of control. The name felt like a bitter joke. What justice exists in decisions made by faceless bureaucrats who have never looked into the eyes of the people they detain—who never hear our voices or witness our growth?

It was now painfully clear that my consultant had no real authority. Though Dr. Dickson was professional and polite, his role was more messenger than decision-maker. His reports were filtered through the Ministry's lens—stripped of nuance, context, and humanity.

I had done everything asked of me. I was stable. I was compliant. I was mobile and motivated. But in their eyes, I was still a risk. Still defined by a moment in time. Still tethered to a diagnosis rather than seen as a whole person.

The punishment was no longer just about what had happened in the past. It was about the ongoing weight of stigma—the way it clung to me like a second skin.

Turning Pain Into Purpose

That evening, I couldn't sleep. I lay in bed with a hollow ache in my chest. Then, I reached for my laptop and began to write. If the system would not let me speak in court, I would speak through my story.

Despite the disappointment, something shifted in me. My determination hardened into resolve. I would return to my family—not broken, but whole, and with my voice intact.

In my search for community, I discovered the *Mental Health Justice Network*. It felt like a lifeline—a space where stories like mine weren't dismissed, but honoured. I subscribed and became an active member, not just as a survivor, but as a nurse with a story that could no longer be silenced.

Through this network, I began connecting with others who believed—as I did—that emotional trauma deserves legal recognition. I reached out to advocacy groups, engaged in forums, and slowly built relationships with people who truly understood the pain of institutionalisation and the deep-rooted injustices baked into the system.

I realised I wanted to use my voice not only to tell my story, but to support and educate others—especially fellow nurses who felt isolated, targeted, or voiceless within the NHS. If my experience could help even one person feel less alone, then it mattered.

This chapter in my journey is not just about reclaiming justice. It is about reclaiming identity. Dignity. Truth.

Before the forced Clopixol injection, I never imagined that one day I would become a patient in the very system I once served with pride. As a nurse trained in Africa, I came to the UK with dreams of healing, helping, and building a better life. I did not expect to encounter a wall of suspicion and silence—not from patients, but from colleagues.

When I was most vulnerable, I was not offered compassion. I was restrained, misdiagnosed, and forcibly medicated. My voice—the very essence of my profession—was taken from me.

Chapter Ten:

From Survivor to Advocate

"Your story is the key that can unlock someone else's prison."

Publishing my first book marked a turning point. For the first time since my ordeal began, I felt in control of my own story. The silence that had once smothered me was finally broken. What began as a deeply personal act of survival became a public declaration of resistance — and, unexpectedly, a source of connection.

I deliberately chose the provocative title *White English Nurses Eat African Nurses* to spark conversation. I knew it would outrage some and validate others. I wanted Black and foreign-trained nurses — those who had also endured silencing and betrayal — to read it and say, *"You told my story too."* That, for me, would be the moment the book stopped being just about me. It would become a mirror for many, and a challenge to a profession that has long ignored its complicity in systemic harm.

Through the Mental Health Justice Network, I began participating in webinars and online forums. I shared my story not just as a psychiatric survivor, but as a nurse who had seen the system from both sides of the bedrail. I began writing articles and short reflections, contributing to conversations about institutional racism, emotional trauma, and the ethics of forced treatment.

I knew it wouldn't be easy. There would be backlash — professional, legal, even personal. But I reminded myself: the cost of silence had already been too high.

At the same time, I vowed never to stop reflecting on my identity as a nurse. I am not alone in feeling betrayed by a profession that taught compassion but tolerated cruelty. I want to help create spaces where nurses — especially those from migrant or minoritised backgrounds — can speak freely, seek support, and find solidarity.

This chapter of my life is not without pain. But it is also filled with purpose. I am no longer just a patient. I am no longer just a victim.

I am a witness.
I am still a nurse.

Chapter Eleven:

Conclusion: Speaking the Unspoken

"What we don't need in the midst of struggle is shame for being human."
— BRENÉ BROWN

As I write this final chapter, I look back not only on what I endured, but on what I survived—and transformed.

This point was not reached suddenly. It is the result of years—decades—of carrying burdens in silence. As a Black African woman, a mother, and a nurse, I had learned to wear strength like armour. I built a life on care, discipline, and resilience. But underneath that exterior was someone who had never been allowed to fully fall apart, to grieve properly, or to speak honestly about pain.

In the healthcare profession, we are trained to look after others, to suppress our own struggles in service of those in need. I had always been the caregiver. But who cares for the caregiver when she is the one unraveling? Who listens when the strong become fragile?

This book is not a confession. It is a declaration. A declaration that mental illness does not discriminate. That trauma—especially when unacknowledged—can push even the most composed among us to the edge. It is also a reflection on how culture, stigma, and silence can become barriers to healing—particularly for African women taught to endure rather than express.

My story is painful, but it is also one of survival. It is about rediscovering parts of myself that were lost long before that darkest day. In writing this, I reclaim my voice. And in sharing it, I hope to reach others—patients, professionals, mothers, daughters, anyone—who may be suffering in silence, believing they are alone.

If you are reading this, perhaps you too are looking for understanding, or for hope. I want you to know that even at your lowest point, you are still worthy of healing. This is the beginning of my truth. And maybe, in it, you will find pieces of your own.

Through this journey, I have come to understand that my healing cannot depend solely on what the system offers—or withholds. Healing has come through reclaiming my story, publishing my truth, building alliances, and standing beside others who refuse to be silenced.

There are still many unanswered questions. There is still no legal redress for the trauma I suffered. But I am no longer waiting for the system to validate my experience. I am part of a movement now—of survivors, truth-tellers, and mental health justice advocates.

I offer this book to the nurse who feels voiceless. To the patient afraid no one will believe them. To the professional gaslit by a system that claims to "care." To the grieving families still waiting for answers. And to anyone who has ever felt broken by the very structures meant to help them heal.

Let this be the beginning of a broader conversation.

Let this be one more step toward truth, accountability, and reform.

And let this book be proof:
Even in silence, you are not alone.
Even in pain, your story matters.
Even after everything—you can rise.

Epilogue:

The Journey Continues

"You may not control all the events that happen to you, but you can decide not to be reduced by them."
— MAYA ANGELOU

Healing is not a destination. It is a path I walk every day—with every breath, every memory, every act of courage to speak when silence feels safer.

Since writing this book, I have continued to grow into a new version of myself—not defined by diagnosis, stigma, or the cruelty I endured, but by the strength I've reclaimed. I am now part of a wider network of survivors, nurses, advocates, and reformers who believe in the power of lived experience to change systems.

I still carry the wounds, but I also carry wisdom. I know that vulnerability is not weakness, and telling the truth—especially when it is inconvenient—is an act of justice.

This memoir began as a lifeline. It has become a lantern.

If you are someone still navigating the shadows, I offer this light to you. If you are part of the system, I ask you to listen—truly listen—to those your policies and practices affect. And if you have ever doubted your right to speak your truth, let this book be your permission.

The journey continues—not just for me, but for all of us working toward a world where care means compassion, not control.

Acknowledgements

To my family—especially my husband and children—thank you for your unwavering love, your patience, and your belief in me even when I could not believe in myself. You stood by me through the darkest nights and helped me find my way back to the light.

To my legal team and advocates who fought for my voice when I had none—your work gave me hope. To the few professionals within the system who showed kindness, thank you for reminding me that humanity still exists in healthcare.

To my peers in the ward, thank you for your solidarity, your humour, and your strength. We were not just patients—we were people, and I will never forget the bond we shared.

To the Mental Health Justice Network, and all the survivors who reached out with stories, support, and sisterhood—you helped me realise I was not alone. Your courage helped ignite mine.

To every Black, migrant, or marginalised nurse who has ever felt erased, silenced, or betrayed by the profession they served—this book is for you. I see you. I honour your resilience.

To Christine Pratt and other pioneers who have named the silent epidemic of injustice in mental health—you gave language to pain that too often goes unnamed.

And finally, to the reader—thank you for witnessing this story. Whether you are a survivor, an ally, a professional, or simply someone trying to understand: thank you for listening. May this be the start of more conversations, more truths told, and more systems held to account.

We are still here.
We are still rising.

Appendixes

Appendix One:

Clinical Note on Clopixol and Depression

Clopixol (zuclopenthixol) is a first-generation antipsychotic medication commonly used in the treatment of schizophrenia and other psychotic disorders. It functions primarily through **dopamine D2 receptor antagonism**, leading to decreased dopaminergic activity in the brain's mesolimbic and mesocortical pathways. While this mechanism may be beneficial in managing psychotic symptoms, it can have **deleterious effects** when used inappropriately—particularly in individuals who do not meet the diagnostic criteria for psychosis.

1. Risk of Depressive Decompensation

In individuals with **stress-related disorders, burnout, or trauma**, the blockade of dopamine can suppress motivation, pleasure, and affect regulation. This pharmacological effect may precipitate or worsen:

- **Major depressive symptoms** such as anhedonia, psychomotor retardation, and affective flattening

- **Cognitive impairments**, including slowed thinking and decreased emotional responsiveness
- **Dysphoric reactions**, especially when the patient has not consented to treatment or when trust in the healthcare system has been eroded

2. Akathisia and Suicidality

Clopixol is associated with a high risk of **akathisia**, a form of medication-induced inner restlessness often misinterpreted as agitation or anxiety. Akathisia is a **well-established risk factor for suicidal ideation and behavior**, especially in patients already in psychological distress. In institutional settings, this can be easily overlooked or dismissed as noncompliance or behavioral disturbance.

3. Diagnostic Misapplication

Administering Clopixol **without a comprehensive psychiatric assessment**—as sometimes occurs during emergency detentions under mental health legislation—carries the risk of **diagnostic error**. Presentations of exhaustion, grief, racialized workplace trauma, or adjustment disorder may be misclassified as psychosis, resulting in **iatrogenic harm** from inappropriate antipsychotic treatment.

4. Ethical and Human Rights Considerations

Forced administration of depot antipsychotics, especially in the absence of psychotic features, raises significant **ethical**

and legal concerns. This is particularly urgent when patients report **deterioration in mood, emotional numbing, or suicidal ideation** following treatment. Failure to recognize or document these adverse effects can lead to **systemic neglect of harm**, compromising both safety and recovery.

Conclusion

Clopixol is a potent neuroleptic agent. When used outside of clear psychotic indications, particularly in **vulnerable or misdiagnosed individuals**, it may **induce or exacerbate severe depressive episodes**, increasing the risk of suicide. Mental health professionals are urged to approach its use with **clinical caution**, **cultural sensitivity**, and **trauma-informed awareness**, ensuring that patients' voices and lived experiences are not silenced in the name of treatment.

Appendix Two:

How Clopixol Can Trigger Severe Depression

Clopixol (also known as zuclopenthixol) is a strong antipsychotic drug often used to treat people who are experiencing psychosis—such as hearing voices, paranoia, or extreme confusion. It works by blocking a brain chemical called **dopamine**, which plays a key role in how we feel motivation, pleasure, and emotional connection.

While Clopixol can help some people with psychosis feel more stable, **it can be harmful if given to someone who is not psychotic**—especially if that person is already stressed, grieving, or experiencing trauma. Unfortunately, this happens more often than it should.

Why It Can Make Depression Worse

- **It numbs the brain**: Dopamine is a "feel good" chemical. When it's blocked too much, a person can feel flat, disconnected, hopeless, or like their emotions have been switched off.
- **It causes restlessness and distress**: Clopixol can trigger a side effect called **akathisia**—a horrible feeling of inner

restlessness, panic, or agitation. Some people describe it as feeling like they want to "crawl out of their skin." This side effect is closely linked to **suicidal thoughts**.

- **It dulls thinking and feeling**: The drug can slow down thinking and make it harder to concentrate or make decisions—adding to the emotional weight of depression.
- **It may be used without proper assessment**: Sometimes, especially during mental health crises, people are given Clopixol **without a full evaluation**. If someone is struggling from grief, overwork, trauma, or burnout—not psychosis—this medication can make things **much worse**, not better.

When the System Gets It Wrong

In some cases, people—especially Black patients or immigrants—are **misunderstood or misdiagnosed** in crisis. Their pain or frustration is mistaken for aggression or madness. Instead of receiving care, they are medicated into silence. This is not just a clinical error—it's a form of **systemic injustice** that can deepen suffering.

Why This Matters

If someone begins to feel worse after taking a psychiatric drug, especially if they weren't fully informed or didn't agree to take it, **their experience should be taken seriously**. Mental health treatment should always involve listening, careful diagnosis, and respect for the person's story—not just symptom control.

Final Thought

Drugs like Clopixol can help some people—but they can also **harm others if misused or given without consent**. No one should be forced to take medication that makes them feel worse, especially when they are already vulnerable. Listening, respect, and careful assessment should always come first

Reflection Questions for You

This section is for anyone who has read *After Injection* and wants to reflect more deeply—whether you are a survivor, healthcare worker, student, loved one, or advocate. These questions are here to spark conversation, healing, and change.

You may wish to journal your answers, discuss them with others, or simply sit with them in quiet reflection.

Understanding Mental Health

- Have you or someone close to you ever experienced a mental health crisis? What helped—or failed to help—in that situation?
- What emotions did Angeline's story evoke in you? Did any parts feel familiar, surprising, or uncomfortable?
- Has this book changed the way you understand depression, trauma, or psychosis? In what way?

Speaking About Suicide

- Why do you think suicide is still so hard to talk about openly in many families, cultures, or workplaces?
- What role do shame, silence, or fear play in preventing people from seeking help?

- What would it take to create safer, more compassionate spaces for suicide survivors to be heard?

The Mental Health System

- What thoughts or concerns did you have about Angeline's experience of forced treatment and misdiagnosis?
- In your opinion, what should informed consent and dignity look like in mental healthcare?
- How can professionals better recognize the difference between trauma, stress, and serious mental illness?

Racism, Power, and Systemic Injustice

- How did racism and institutional bias affect Angeline's journey through the healthcare and legal systems?
- Have you ever witnessed or experienced discrimination in healthcare or the workplace? What was the impact?
- What changes would you want to see in the NHS or mental health system to better support Black women, immigrants, and other marginalized communities?

Healing and Purpose

- What does recovery mean to you? Is it just surviving—or finding meaning after the pain?
- How can storytelling, writing, or speaking out help transform suffering into strength?
- What is one small action you can take—to reduce stigma, support a loved one, or speak out against injustice?

"To heal is not to erase the past, but to give it meaning."

www.ingramcontent.com/pod-product-compliance
Ingram Content Group UK Ltd.
Pitfield, Milton Keynes, MK11 3LW, UK
UKHW022046241025
8589UKWH00004B/563

9 781036 922306